Fighting a Losing Battle

How I Lost 100 Lbs. in Ten Months

Robertrese Allen

ISBN 978-1-64003-946-9 (Paperback)
ISBN 978-1-64003-947-6 (Digital)

Copyright © 2018 Robertrese Allen
All rights reserved
First Edition

All rights reserved. No part of this publication may be reproduced, distributed, or transmitted in any form or by any means, including photocopying, recording, or other electronic or mechanical methods without the prior written permission of the publisher. For permission requests, solicit the publisher via the address below.

Covenant Books, Inc.
11661 Hwy 707
Murrells Inlet, SC 29576
www.covenantbooks.com

Contents

Acknowledgments 5

Introduction: It's A Fixed Fight!........................7

Chapter 1: Transformation 13

Chapter 2: Begin with the End in "Mind".......21

Chapter 3: Water Works...................................29

Chapter 4: The Great Plateau 34

Chapter 5: To Eat or to Not Eat 46

Chapter 6: Brand-New You—How Does It Feel?...........51

Acknowledgments

> But thou, O LORD, [art] a shield for me; my glory, and the lifter up of mine head. (Ps. 3:3, KJV)

I'd be remiss if I didn't first acknowledge my Lord and Savior, Christ Jesus! Lord, you are my everything! Thank you for loving me and believing in me. Thank you for healing me and blessing me to be an example to all who read this book.

To my husband and best friend, Theodore Allen Jr., I love you more than words can say. You saw what I couldn't see. And you loved me through it. Your love and support through the years has been the wind beneath my wings. I love you.

To my children, Danyel Curry (Martavius), Dapheni Allen, Daniel Allen, DeMarcus Allen, and my grandchildren Morgan and Alexander Curry, I love each of you with all of my heart. You are my reason for living. I'm so proud to be your mother, mother in love, and grandmother!

To my Father, Robert J. Henderson. I'm so grateful for your weekly advice and wisdom. Thank you for loving me unconditionally. I love you with all my heart. I'll always be Daddy's little girl!

To all of my family, friends, and colleagues. Thank you for your support and for believing in me. I love you to pieces!

Introduction

It's A Fixed Fight!

I want to jump ahead to the end of our story. A spoiler of sorts. I want you to know that *you win*! After reading this book, you will no longer have a fear or concern of not being able to lose weight and keep it off. The things that have been holding you back will no longer have power over you. You'll master both the psychology and science of true weight loss. You are destined for greatness. Your weight loss victory is just one proof of that. You can enjoy a life full of health and vitality beyond your wildest dreams!

If you're like me, you've read and tried a lot of things. I'll tell you now—the difference maker for me was the *action* that I took. I got sick and tired of losing, and you must do the same. Your actions will determine your outcome. Decide right now to *act*.

From the beginning, my intent is to be a blessing to all who read this book. In my heart, the best way to do so is to be very transparent and truthful. So let's get started.

The following words taunted me for years: fat, big, thick, overweight, obese, unhappy, unfit, inferior, insecure. I've felt or experienced these words in some shape or form over the past twenty years. In my mind, I entertained presumptions of what the opinions of others were of me. I had a lot of help. Family assumes you're depressed and unhappy. Friends don't mention it but wonder what's going on with you. Others presume you inferior or beneath them because of how you look, knowing nothing about your character and who you are inside. Even though I dealt with these negative thoughts, I've always portrayed a happy exterior. People naturally assume if you're overweight, you are unhappy. But if you're happy and bubbly, like me, they question how you could be. "How can she be so happy?" The answer was simple. I chose to be happy! Regardless of what I was dealing with, I chose to be happy.

Sidebar: Happiness is a choice. Happiness is a weapon against depression and low self-esteem!

Sometimes, I'd wonder: Does anyone truly know me? Why can't they see what I see? My answer was clear. They just couldn't! It was not for them to see; I had to see. I say the same for you. As long as you can see and visualize your desired outcome, you can be it, have it, and achieve it. I eventually concluded that everyone had their own opinions and theories about why I had gained so much weight. I'm speaking of those who knew me from before. How they interacted with me was based on how they felt about me.

In my younger years, I didn't have a weight issue. I have four wonderful children, and they didn't cause me to gain weight either. It was never a concern to me until after age thirty. Once I started to gain weight, a whole new era of challenges began. Deep down, I felt that it was coming. I thought there had to be a reason for it. When I was around thirty-six years old, I remember waking up out of my sleep from what I concluded to be a terrible nightmare. In my dream, I saw myself lying across my bed, crying. I was crying because I was three hundred pounds! I never told anyone about the dream. I dismissed it and said that would never happen.

I'd been slim, average sized, my whole life so that wouldn't happen to me. But it did happen! Not suddenly. I put the pounds on gradually. Pound for pound. Year after year. Slowly yet consistently, my weight increased. Oh, believe me, throughout my twenty-plus-year weight-gain war, I had many battles! Diets after diets. Fasting and praying. Eating healthy. Or so I thought. The weight kept coming. Yes, I'd exercise and see a little progress. It would be great for a while. Then over time, I'd break my regimen, and the weight would come right back. Sounds familiar? Eventually, I concluded this was it. I'm supposed to be this size. Keep in mind I dreamt it years ago. So somewhere in the back of my mind, I allowed the seed of that dream to become my reality.

For the thing which I greatly feared
is come upon me, and that which I
was afraid of is come unto me.

—Job 3:25, KJV

To be quite honest, for years, I tried to dismiss that dream. But the underlying fear of it being real made me accept it as my fate; I guess. The "losing battle" was going on in my head long before it manifested on the outside. I believed in the possibility of the dream being real because I am a dreamer. Everybody dreams, right? Let me be more precise. Certain dreams I'd have would stand out. Not your "average busy mind" or "had too much pizza last night" kind of dream. I know that sounds weird, but I have had several dreams to come to pass in my lifetime. Very specific dreams. For example, I had three consecutive dreams about having twin girls. I was sixteen at the time, cheerleading and running cross-country and track. Babies were the last thing on my mind!

In the first dream, I saw myself holding to babies in my arms and wearing canary yellow. I heard myself asking, "Whose babies are these?" No kidding! In the second dream, these babies were dressed in powder blue. I asked, "Are they boys or girls?" In the third dream, I saw toddler girls! I knew then that they were mine and what their names would be. Well, guess what? They are thirty years old now!

I can't explain it, but certain dreams would leave me pondering for days, months, and like this weight-gain dream, for years. Even though I tried to fight it, subconsciously, I called that dream to mind every time I gained more weight. I realize now that I didn't have to succumb to that dream. All I had to do was face my fear, believe, and see a different outcome. Believe in something better. Believe in my God. Believe in myself. You get the point.

My hope as you read this book is that you rid yourself of all limiting beliefs as it relates to you losing weight. You are already victorious. Now let's just point out some practical strategies to help you along your journey.

Enjoy,
Robertrese

Chapter 1

Transformation

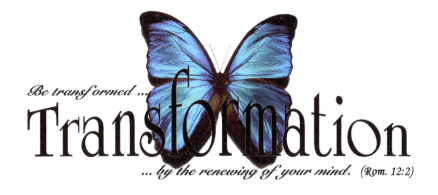

Transformation—are you ready for yours? This book will empower you. It will also challenge you to get out of your comfort zone. Our first step is *honesty*. So let's be honest. What you have been doing up to this point hasn't worked. You've got to decide to change. You must allow change. It all begins with a decision. Long before you see your desired results on the outside, you must first see them inside. There has to be an inward transformation.

The Butterfly Effect

Have you ever studied the butterfly? What it has to endure before becoming the beautiful creation we love to see. How it starts from a low state, crawling around as a caterpillar, a potential victim of their environment. You know, bird food! How it elevates itself to a higher state of living and then literally surrounds itself with what it needs to grow and transform. How when inside of the cocoon, it goes through an amazing transformation. Butterflies have to shed some old stuff and embrace new ideals—literally die to self in order to become something beautiful and great! See, the caterpillar knows that it's destined to become a butterfly. Those ideals were implanted in them by their Creator. As a result, we get to see what they become. Amazing, right?

In a lot of ways, we are like that butterfly. We too must change and surround ourselves with the right elements to become what we were created to be. First, by acknowledging where you are. Be truthful with yourself—face yourself. I know that can be a scary thought, but you cannot master what you will not confront. Being honest with yourself about where you are is crucial. Transformation begins inwardly long before any outward manifestation appears. Make no mistake about it. It begins in the deep places of your inward being. It begins with your thoughts. Romans 12:2 tells us that we will be transformed by the "renewing" of our minds. In other words, you must change your thinking before your actions will change.

You might ask, "Change my thinking about what?" About yourself. Perhaps about the possibility of losing weight once and for all. Your thoughts are so powerful. Whatever you think, you say. Whatever you say, you believe. Whatever you believe, you act out. I had to think my way to health, wellness, happiness, and peace. I had to become intimate with my body inside and out, and that's a point to note. <u>Getting to know yourself is also key to your success. Your body is your gift. Study your body. Listen to what your body tells you. Pay attention!</u>

It's Okay to Ask God for Help

And this is the confidence that we have in him that, if we ask any thing according to his will, he heareth us: And if we know that he hear us, whatsoever we ask, we know that we have the petitions that we desired of him

—1 John 5:14, KJV

If you could do it own your own, it would already be done. Rid yourself of all pride. Ask for help, and not just from anybody. Ask the one who created you. As with anything you have success with in life, you're bound to be asked by some, "How did you do it?" or "What are you doing?" In my case, I've been asked a little bit of both, so I began to really think about my answers. There were a number of things I could attribute to my success, but the first of these was *prayer*. Now to be perfectly honest, I didn't want to pray at first. In my heart, I didn't want to "bother" the Lord with something so petty. Something that I could handle on my own, or so I thought. I'm sure there are others of you out there that thought just like me. You know, go to God with the big problems, not the petty stuff like losing weight. Then I realized. God cares about *all* of me! Why shouldn't I talk to him about my petty stuff? After all, he took the time to number the hairs on my head (Matt. 10:30). I'm pretty sure he wants me to look and feel good.

Therefore, I got out of my own way and simply asked for his help. I asked according to his Word, with the confidence that he was listening to me and that he loved me. Then I went on my merry way with the determination that I was about to lose those unwanted pounds.

You see, nothing will manifest in your life that you don't first accept as *truth*. I had to believe that I could change my situation. As a matter of fact, it was changed already. I just had to see it. We'll talk about that a little later in the book.

Don't let fear conquer you.

If you recall earlier, I exposed a secret fear that I suppressed for twenty-plus years—the fear of weighing three hundred pounds. Well, now let me tell you how I conquered that fear. It wasn't pretty, but it was certainly worth it. Here's the short version:

January 2016, I had a really bad toothache in my upper right molar. I finally went to my dentist only to be told she couldn't pull my tooth because my blood pressure was too high. I frantically denied having high blood pressure, but the numbers were the numbers. I can recall having chronic headaches for a few weeks. I assumed my headaches were a result of my toothache, so I went to my doctor and they confirmed, yep, high blood pressure. Not only that, but they forced me to get on the scale! OMG! Get on the scale? Really? That was one giant I really didn't want to face, but I did. My weight was 309 pounds!

All kinds of thoughts were running through my mind. The dream had come true! When? Where? How? This was the worst day of my life, it seemed. All the negative feelings seemed to rush in on me at once. It took all that was in me to hold back the tears. Once I calmed down, I remembered my prayer asking God for help, and he answered my prayer. I didn't like the answer I received, but I quickly resolved that something had to change!

Well, the first step to change is acknowledging where you are. I had to face it before I could change it. I had to run toward that which I had feared for so many years. This was the next step to my transformation, confronting my fear. You cannot conquer what you will not confront! I was in unfamiliar territory. Again, I didn't grow up with a weight problem nor high blood pressure. I was pretty much slim all my life, even after having four children by age twenty-nine. So these consequences of gaining weight had the potential of spinning me into a downward spiral. Nevertheless, I took it all in and made the decision, once again, to change!

I tried the prescribed meds for a month, but they made me sicker, so I realized I had to "wean" myself back to good health. Although I have great respect for doctors, I refused to let them get me hooked on medication. I made the decision to pay the price for restored health. Part of this price was weaning myself. In other words, I had thought myself to good health (be intentional). I had to abort my bad eating habits. They were literally killing me. I had to start paying attention to how my body acted to certain foods, so must you. Remember, your body is your gift.

Whatever You Think about the Most, You Attract

I had to "discipline" my thoughts. I had to begin with the end in mind. In other words, I had to see the best version of myself in my mind and work toward it, and this wasn't easy. However, you must believe against all odds. Think about what you want, not what you don't want. Thoughts become things. Thoughts are unspoken words. Thoughts create vision, good or bad. Your mind is very powerful. What you constantly think about will manifest in your life. Sure, my faith was challenged. There were some nights that I cried all night long. My pillow was drenched with tears because I felt so helpless. Eventually, I got stronger.

FIGHTING A LOSING BATTLE

Finally, brethren, whatsoever things are true, whatsoever things are honest, whatsoever things are just, whatsoever things are pure, whatsoever things are lovely, whatsoever things are of good report; if [there be] any virtue, and if there be any praise, think on these things.

—Philippians 4:8, KJV

I lost twenty-five pounds from February to March of 2016—mostly water. I had begun consuming at least one-half gallon of water per day at this point. There are so many benefits to drinking water. We'll get into that later, but make a mental note: *to help you lose weight, you must drink 50 percent of your weight in ounces of water per day.* It works!

Affirmations

Seeding your subconscious mind with good things are crucial to your success. Affirmations are one of the best ways to plant good *"seed"* in your subconscious. Your thought life produces after its own kind. Bad thoughts produce bad results; good thoughts, good results. So accept as truth that thoughts are things, and thoughts bring results. Affirmations help to discipline your thought life. Say them out loud. Affirmations like: *I am healthy. I am strong. Good things are happening to me now. I am victorious. I am happy. I am a delight for all to see. I am my perfect size. I feel great. I am a blessing to others.*

At first, it will seem crazy and weird. You will have conflict in your thinking. But the more you say things you want, the faster they will become your reality. Say the right things over and over until *you* believe them. Once you believe, they happen.

This is what I did and continue to do. Every week, I begin to see results. I'd lose two pounds, three pounds, sometimes five pounds!

Chapter 2

Begin with the End in "Mind"

Praise Him in Advance

I remember thinking, "Lord, I asked for help, but I didn't want to be sick!" In my heart of heart, I knew it wasn't God's doing. I just had to battle some personal demons. Let me add this nugget: The quickest way out of your trial is to praise your way out! Wake up every morning with thanksgiving in your heart and speak words of praise out of your mouth. *Be intentional.*

Speaking positive words out of your mouth every morning will set the tone for a very successful day. Your words program your subconscious, so be careful of what you say!

Now I left off in the previous chapter talking about the power of your mind. I'd like now to suggest some things to you. First, what you believe will determine your actions and ultimately, your outcome. You have both a conscious mind and a subconscious mind. They must be in agreement for you to achieve your desired results. Look at this picture. What does it show you?

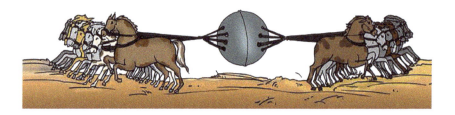

Can you see that if the horses pull in opposite directions, the ball goes nowhere? This is exactly what happens when our conscious mind tries to go somewhere that the subconscious mind doesn't agree with.

What you believe to be true, what you truly believe, gets embedded in your subconscious mind. Your mind must be in total agreement.

You have to begin with your end result "in mind." See yourself healthy. Post pictures up of how you want to look. *Say to yourself repeatedly, "I am healthy," "I am my perfect size," "I am beautiful," "I am a healthy weight," "I am in perfect health," "I am more than able."* Get the picture?

FIGHTING A LOSING BATTLE

Thou shall decree a thing, and it shall be established unto thee: And the Light shall shine upon thy ways.

—Job 22:28

Let me reiterate. What you say over and over again will seed your subconscious mind. Your subconscious mind takes its orders from what you speak out loud, and it will find a way to make it come to pass. Whatever you say is a command. Start your statements with *I am, I will, I can, I have*. Your thoughts and your words have power. Pay attention to what you think and say.

Someone may be reading and asking, "What does this have to do with me losing weight?" My answer to you is *everything*! Visualization, seeding, and affirmations are powerful weapons to your success. You can try every diet and weight loss plan known to man, but until you believe in your heart of hearts that you can lose weight, you won't. So begin with a clear picture of what success is for you. Don't compare yourself with anyone else. Please, please don't do that. For me, being a size 14 is great. I don't care to be any smaller. To each his or her own. You decide. You determine what size or weight will be the best version of yourself. Write it down. Speak it out loud. Then work your way to it. Remember, the choice is yours!

What Gets Measured Gets Improved

My mentor in business is known for making the statement above. For years, he's coached my husband and myself with this philosophy. In short, you have to keep a track record. Whether good or bad, high or low, you have to measure your results, or the lack thereof. You have to monitor your activity, make the necessary changes in behavior, and your success will be eminent.

I applied this principle to my eating habits. In my opinion, there are no such things as diets. Instead, I call them lifestyle changes. To me, a diet is temporal. It's short term, something you attempt to do in order to get into that dress for your class reunion, or that wedding dress or tuxedo. Maybe you've planned a vacation for the summer and want that beach body. Get my drift? But the "diet" mindset is temporary. It causes you to yo-yo diet. You may reach your goal. However, after the "event" is over, you return to your old way of eating until the next big event in your life, thus repeating the cycle of gaining and losing weight. It's an emotional roller coaster that I refuse to ride again! Weight loss requires a lifestyle change. It's permanent.

Good Measure

At first, I loathed the change. It didn't feel good at all! But I knew that if I didn't change my actions, my outcome would not change. There were three main areas I knew I needed to "measure" in my eating habits. *I needed to measure my salt intake, my sugar intake, and my water intake.* These new daily disciplines were the secrets to my success.

The idea of reading food labels and not being able to eat what I wanted because it was either too high in sodium or sugar seemed dreadful at the beginning. But now looking back, I am so glad I did!

Most of the foods we buy are processed foods and loaded with sodium. Foods high in sodium and high in sugar, frankly, are not good for your health. You have to start paying attention to what you are putting in your body.

How Much Sodium or Sugar Should I Have a Day

The American Heart Association recommends no more than 2,300 milligrams a day. But for adults, *an ideal limit of no more than 1,500 milligrams per day.*

To give you a sodium shocker, do you know how much sodium is in one slice of cheese pizza? Five hundred milligrams! The amounts are greater when you add meats and veggies. What about that quarter pounder from McDonald's? It's 1,090 milligrams! This used to be my favorite. Notice I said *used to be*! You can google the *nutritional values of all your favorite foods and restaurants,* and you'll be unpleasantly surprised at the results! Too much sodium is dangerous for your health, and it's one of the root causes of obesity and high blood pressure. You have got to measure your sodium intake. It's not hard, and it will force you to change what you eat.

What about Sugar?

How many grams of sugar should you consume in a day? The American Heart Association recommends most

American women *eat* to no more than 100 calories *per day* of *sugar* (six teaspoons or 20 grams) and that men eat no more than 150 calories *per day* (or about nine teaspoons or 36 grams).

As you can imagine, this is going to be a real shocker to your body. In our society, with all the fast-food restaurants around, we'll go over these limits daily. You have to measure your sodium and sugar intakes. You also have to measure your water intake. We'll take about it in the next chapter.

Bad Measure

I want to stress the negative consequences of having a high sodium and high sugar diet. Fast foods are loaded with salt, and Americans eat a lot of fast food. I'm not saying all salt is bad. I am saying, however, that too much salt is bad for you. Eat at home more. High salt intake causes your body to retain extra water, which increases your blood pressure levels. High blood pressure can lead to all kinds of illnesses and diseases such as heart attacks and strokes. Likewise, the same dangers can happen with too much sugar in your diet; it is life threatening. *Eating and drinking too much sugar* causes weight gain, abdominal obesity, elevated blood *sugar*, and high blood pressure. I'm being redundant on purpose!

Most people don't believe me when I tell them this, so I have to show them the photo below. My sugar levels spiked from 78 in February 2016 to *841* in March 2016! Due in part to, in my opinion, new medications prescribed to me for high blood pressure. This medication literally dehydrated me and caused me to experience horrific side effects. I was so scared. At times, my heart would race at rapid speeds. I would become delusional. My vision became very, very blurry to the point that I couldn't work or even drive. I feared losing my eyesight. Obviously, I stopped taking the medicine! My traumatic experience forced me to make the changes. Although unpleasant, I'm truly thankful to God for all of the knowledge I gained and, most of all, that it didn't kill me!

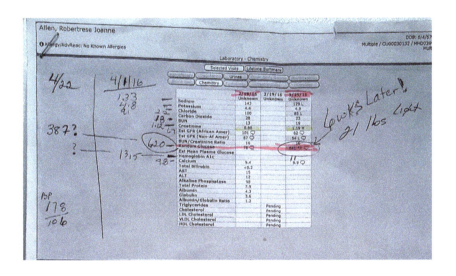

What Did I Do to Counteract

Drink water! Our body tries to naturally dilute itself by retaining water when there is too much salt in our system. Drinking water flushes out toxins brought in by too much salt and sugar, so drinking water will literally save your life. It did mine! Praise God!

Try this. For the next seven days, drink only water, then measure your results afterward. You'll be amazed! Now let's talk more about water.

Chapter 3

Water Works

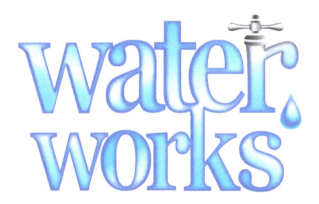

This may be the shortest chapter in my book. However, it's the most important one there is. *Water works*! It's amazing how many people, when I tell them what I did to lose weight, hit me with the statements: "I hate drinking water" or "I don't drink water"! A shocking number of people have the same sentiment. I think it's because we've been "sugared" to death—*literally*. The craving for something sweet to drink all the time has caused us as a nation to become morbidly obese. We drink soda like water, and we've lost a love for the most valuable, most necessary beverage for the human body. You guessed it—*water!*

Water Facts

Did you know that the amount of water in the human body ranges from 50–75 percent?

According to the Mayo Clinic, our bodies are about 60 percent water. Whatever percentage is the most accurate, would you agree that we are mostly water? Water is the most vital part of our makeup. It regulates our body temperature and flushes waste from our bodies, as we mentioned before. Water is what makes our bodies work. Did you also know that our major organs are predominately water? Our lungs are 90 percent water. Our brain is 70 percent. Our blood is 80 percent water. So why drink water? Really?

Well, outside of the obvious facts mentioned above, you literally cannot live without it! As a matter of fact, the average person cannot survive going three days without water. Water is a large percentage of our makeup. Without it, we die.

How Much Water Should You Drink?

Half of your body weight in ounces. Now there's a lot of debate about the amounts and the types of water to drink. To save myself a lot of typing, I'll just tell you what worked and is working for me. I chose to drink alkaline water. As I mentioned earlier, I had to measure three main things in my diet: my sodium intake, my sugar intake, and my water intake.

I found out the benefits of drinking alkaline water. Here are a few:
1. helps fight disease,
2. boost immune system,
3. promotes healthy pH in the body,
4. neutralizes acid in the blood stream,
5. helps with weight loss.

Again, these were some of my reasons. As I increased my water intake, I felt better. The swelling in my hands and feet went away, almost instantly. I began averaging at least 3 pounds a week in weight loss. Obviously, that excess water was stored because of too much salt in my diet. I found out something I didn't know. Drinking water *helps maintain the balance of body fluids*. The functions of these bodily fluids include digestion, circulation, creation of saliva, sending nutrients, and regulation of our body temperature.

Through what's called our posterior pituitary gland, our brain communicates with our kidneys and tells it how much water to excrete as urine or hold on to for reserves. In simple terms, my body was holding on to fluid because I wasn't drinking enough water. The same may be the case with you. As I mentioned earlier, a lot of people don't like to drink water. Some complain of going to the bathroom too much. Well, your body has to dump all the excess. I felt the same at first, but as my body adjusted, so did my bladder. I also found out that one cause of high blood pressure was dehydration. Once I got this revelation, I really started drinking the proper amount of water. I read an article by Gloria Donaldson, "This Is What Happens When You Drink Only Water for 30 Days", and it confirmed everything I was experiencing. I encourage you to google it for yourself. Here are the main points I took from it: 1) When water is your only beverage for a long period of time, it heals your body! 2) Water flushes out toxins from your vital organs. Thus, causing you to lose weight and crave less sugar.

Once you begin your water regimen, after about a week, other drinks will be less desirable. Try it for one week, then two weeks. Those of you who are really ready for change, try it for thirty days and see what happens! Water is the *key* to weight loss. I can't stress it enough. *Drink water!*

It all started to make sense to me. Without water, our bodies can't function properly. Major transformation occurred as I created my water-drinking discipline. The weight loss was dramatic. I started taking a lot of selfies and posted them on my Facebook page. After a short while, the phone calls started coming in. "What are you doing?" my friends would ask. I'd simply give my three-things version.

Reduce sodium, sugar, and increase water intake. I've heard so many testimonials of others increasing their water intake and getting great results. My mother-in-law began drinking the alkaline water and her blood pressure levels dropped significantly to the point that her doctor asked her what she was doing. My godmother was having trouble with her back, but once she got regimented on water consumption, she too had favorable results. My point is *water works*!

By December 2016 (from February to December), I had lost 104 pounds!

For years, I wondered what was going on with my body—why I looked so "puffy." So the fact that increasing my water intake brought so many health benefits to me, well, let's just say I'm speechless. I am so thankful and grateful to be able to tell my story to my friends and loved ones. If I can do it, anybody can! After ten months of transformation both mentally and physically, I had to face another truth. I needed an exercise regimen!

Now these were like curse words to me! I was too lazy to exercise. Notice I said "was." Present day, I feel horrible if I don't exercise. I started going to my neighborhood recreational center three days a week just to walk on the treadmill for thirty minutes. That was all I was willing to do. After all, my twin daughters had me so regimented on meal prepping, reading food labels, taking my vitamins, I needed to call something on my own. So I'd walk about a mile in thirty minutes, three days a week. Then something happened—I started enjoying it! Oh my, did my competitive juices start to flow. I went from barely doing a mile in thirty minutes to two miles in under thirty minutes, timing myself and taking selfies after each work out (LOL). Gotta love it. So all the pieces of my health puzzle were coming together. Success was mine, but it all began with my mindset. As my thoughts improved, my words improved. As my words improved, my actions improved. And yes, as my actions improved, my results improved. I hope it's sinking in.

Chapter 4

The Great Plateau

The word *plateau* is defined as a "period" of no growth or progress.

There may be times when you feel that you aren't seeing any results. You may ask, "How do I keep from getting stuck?" Well. the short answer is, "Consistency beats spectacular." Just stay true to your regimen and you will see consistent results.

In my opinion, when you think *diet*, you're thinking *temporary*. Which is better? Adding a large log to a fire that is already burning or adding small portions of wood a little at a time? Obviously, the latter, right? Make lifestyle changes. Making small but consistent changes to your diet are more effective and permanent than crash dieting. Crash dieting can lead to all kinds of health consequences. Plus, you're guaranteed to gain the weight back and then some. Broaden your food choices. As I stated from the beginning, become intimate with your body. Pay attention to how your body reacts to the foods you eat. Find a better way to enjoy the foods you love, then enjoy them! Maintaining a consistent regimen is key to not yo-yoing in your diet. You've got to create a regimen. For me, *I had to think of the foods I loved and find a healthy version of them.* I even found new foods that I really enjoyed eating, and water was such a vital part of my process; I don't go a day without it.

However, I can recall at one point getting on the scale and not seeing change. At the time, I felt the need to lose a few more pounds, but it wasn't happening. Then after a while, I'd fluctuate in my weight. I became frustrated because I wanted to lose more weight and certainly didn't want to regain any weight. It seemed the more I focused on the negative, the harder it got.

What's the Worst That Can Happen?

I took a chill pill, or so I told myself. I stopped getting on the scale. Remember, it was frustrating me. After all, I looked great. I felt great. "Just enjoy your victory," I would tell myself. My 80/20 motto stayed in my head. As long as I stayed true to it, I was fine. But there's a danger in becoming too complacent.

Stay True to You

Eventually, I stopped going to the gym. I let any and everything break my focus and my regimen. Little by little, I would eat something I knew wasn't good for me. "I'll do better tomorrow" was the lie that kept me from sticking to a good regimen. After a few months, I noticed certain clothing getting "snug" on me. "Wait just one minute!" I'd shout aloud in my head. My enemy was planning a subtle take over. The weight was coming back, little by little, inch by inch, pound by pound. I flirted with that old unhealthy lifestyle, and I eventually reverted to it. My enemy was my "inner me!" I was losing my grip on a victory that I worked so hard for. Lord, have mercy!

It got harder and harder to resist certain food cravings. Still, I was in denial. "Didn't matter that the scale was weighing in higher. I still look good and can still wear my clothes" is what I'd say to pacify myself.

But things were trending in the wrong direction. I started noticing my lack of desire to drink water. Me? The water queen? Yes! From there, my worst fear gripped me. "I'm gaining the weight back!" "Oh, no!" "I'm almost finished with this book. I can't lose my battle!" "What will people think?" Oh yeah, the fear of the opinions of people tried to take me out. I began noticing little subliminal comments of those around me that didn't say outright but hinted at me gaining weight. I think some hoped I did! LOL. But I quickly concluded my enemy, again, was my inner me.

Thou delivered me from the strivings of the people.
—Psalm 18:43

Side note: you can't live your life worrying about what other people think. People are influenced by circumstances.

If you do well, they praise you. If you do bad, they criticize you. We all have those tendencies. Truth is no one can make you feel inferior without your permission. It's what you say to yourself that matters. I was saying the wrong things to myself. I was focusing on the negative and not the positive, so I had to have a paradigm shift—think the right thoughts.

You create your world with your thoughts and your words. Success is 90 percent mental and 10 percent action!

Remember earlier when I said thoughts were things that produced words that force us to act, and depending on those actions, we fail or we have success.

What you feed your subconscious mind will manifest in your life. There she goes again with that "thinking" stuff. Yep, there I go. Because our thoughts run our life.

I'm spending a lot of time here because this is where the real battle is. Joyce Meyer wrote a book called *Battlefield of the Mind*. I encourage you to get it and read it. It is important for you to understand that you win first in your mind. Then your body will follow. Change your mind-set about weight loss. See it as a natural progression and course in life. *You are healthy, you are wealthy, you are wise. You are attractive. You are a joy for all to see and be around.* Meditate on these words. Say them repeatedly to yourself. You can accomplish great things just with this simple process.

> Be careful what you think, because
> your thoughts run your life.
>
> —Proverbs 4:23, NCV

I shifted my thoughts to my victories, not my failures! I made a list of all the things I had accomplished on my weight loss journey—how I overcame great health challenges, how it felt when I dropped a dress size, then another, and another. Even when times were tough, I recalled my feelings of when I overcame. This is so critical to maintaining our victory over weight loss. If you were like me and gained back some weight that you lost, be encouraged. You will win! Just stay positive and go to war!

Attack the Belly Fat

I've spent a lot of time talking about your mind and how important it is to protect it. Now let me talk about another that needs to be protected. I'm talking about your *core*, your stomach or belly area.

I really hope to amaze you with this knowledge! A healthy belly is key to a healthy body. Most underlying causes of sickness and disease can be traced back to poor digestive health. Ever wonder why no matter what you do, the belly fat won't go away? The problem sometimes lies dormant within your core. Sometimes unknowingly, we do things that cause our bodies to store belly fat. Here are a few examples of things that could be the reason for your unhealthy abdominal area:

1. Chewing Sugar-Free Gum

    Did you know you swallow air while you chew gum and that it becomes trapped in your stomach and small intestines which causes bloating? Sugarless gum is worse because our bodies don't identify with artificial sweeteners. Isn't that crazy?

2. Too Much Stress

    When you're stressed, your body produces a hormone called cortisol. This produces "visceral" fat from other places in your body and stores it in your belly! Solution? Chill out! Avoid stress at all cost. (I noticed this happening to me when I get stressed out in my business.)

3. Not Enough Sleep

    Adults are supposed to sleep at least seven hours every night. Yeah right! But did you know that lack of sleep also increases the cortisol in your body which we know stores belly fat? I also read that lack of sleep increases sugar levels. What?

    I believe that your body naturally heals itself while it's in rest mode. You've got to rest more!

4. Too Much Fiber

    Raffinose is a type of sugar. It is found in vegetables like kale, broccoli, cabbage, and legumes like lentils and peas. Too much causes gas and bloating, so limit your intake of such foods.

5. Constipation

    You've got to drink water. Stay regular. When you're constipated, gas gets trapped behind slow-moving bowels and builds up, causing your belly to swell.

6. Too Much Sodium

    Eating foods that contain a lot of salt can cause your body to retain water and make your stomach look bigger. Your body naturally regulates water retention. As we mentioned is previous chapters, too little water and too much salt can trigger your body to store water.

All of the examples I mentioned can be controlled by you. You can win the belly bulge battle. With some simple tweaks. Let's move on.

A New Way

I spent a lot of time researching what food would be advantageous for my body—for my blood type and health conditions I was challenged with. We'll talk more about those foods in the next chapter. Learning the science of food is truly empowering. You can avoid so many health pitfalls simply by knowing what foods are best for you to eat! However, just knowing these truths was not enough. I had to act on the information I obtained. The same goes for you. You have to apply the knowledge you have to your situation.

I had to do so. Not just one time but over and over again. When I was not doing right, I had to be honest with myself. Let me say, this has been to best antidote to avoiding stagnation: "to thine own self be true." My mother used to quote these words constantly. You have to be truthful with yourself at all times, and you have to practice change.

Change doesn't happen overnight, but consistency will help you achieve the desired results. You are in complete control of what you eat and drink. Master it! If you get off track every now and then, it's okay. Don't punish yourself. That will only make you move more in the direction you don't want to go. Remember, what you focus on grows.

You can avoid what I call the great plateau. Be *intentional* about what you put in your body. Be excited about the lifestyle change, and enjoy your transition. Sometimes, your body gets so used to eating the same foods it adapts and keeps everything level. You may have to throw your body a curve ball. Add a different vegetable; use mustard instead of mayo, and so forth. Add spice and variety every now and then to your eating regimen. Whatever the case, eat to live. Know that the decisions you are making right now will change your life for the better forever.

There Is Something Higher

The things that have pulled you down in life will no longer keep you down. There is a better life in store for you. Remember the butterfly in chapter 1? You've got to get to higher ground. Our failures in life are not designed to keep us down. They come so that we can learn. I learned a lesson of great value. I learned to not take my success for granted. Thank God I did.

I also learned to be patient with myself. To stop being so uptight and in a hurry. Slow, consistent weight loss is *true* weight loss. Be patient.

Do It Again

Here are some tough facts, some hard pills to swallow. If you stop your regimen, if you stop your good eating habits, you will regain the weight. If you try to starve your body (what I call desperation dieting), you will send a signal to your brain to store and reserve fat. Thus, gaining or regaining weight becomes inevitable. If you don't condition your body to rid of stress and toxins through exercising and drinking water, you will keep or regain unwanted weight.

But let patience have her perfect work, that you may be perfect and entire, wanting nothing.

—James 1:4, KJV

You may be asking, "What do I do now?" The answer is simple: *do it again*! Once you know what works, you just simply have to work it. Once you've accomplished something, you can teach it for years. It's like riding a bicycle or driving a car. Once you learn how, it sticks with you for life. You never forget the how-to. Once you know better, you can do better. Knowledge is power. This mindset has been the one thing to help me overcome the fear of regaining the weight that I've lost. Fear and dread are only present in lieu of the unknown; fear tortures you with negative thoughts of what if. What if I gain the weight back? What if I can't maintain the weight loss? What if it was just a fluke?

Faith, on the other hand, asks what-if questions also! What if I lose ten more pounds? How will that look? How will I feel? And so on. Faith and fear are two powerful forces, but they work contrary to one another. Like the illustration I used earlier of the horses pulling in opposite directions. Faith and fear can't work together. The good news is the power to choose is yours! So choose the positive emotions. Choose Faith. Choose Life. Focus on the possibilities of your good dreams coming true. See yourself at the finish line. Keep those feelings at the forefront of your mind. I saw, I felt, I experienced the success of losing one hundred pounds in ten months! In tough times, I would take my mind back to those days, those thoughts of achievement and feeling good. What your "mind" perceives, it will achieve! Don't waste time thinking about the negatives.

Okay, so you fell off the wagon? Get up! Brush yourself off and get going again. Do it again! Do it repeatedly until it becomes second nature to you. Experts say it takes at least twenty-one days to make or break a habit, so get going.

> Finally, brethren, whatsoever things are true, whatsoever things are honest, whatsoever things are just, whatsoever things are pure, whatsoever things are lovely, whatsoever things are of good report; if there be any virtue, and if there be any praise, think on these things.
>
> —Philippians 4:8, KJV

Think on things that you have accomplished in life. As a matter of fact, get a special tablet and write them down. Then when moments of weakness occur, read over them. Remind yourself of the successes you've had. I'm telling you this is so powerful! The power of positive thinking! It's so necessary to helping you get over all weight loss hurdles. So get a vision of yourself in your head of what it looks like when you reach your goal. Burn that image in your mind. How does it feel? What does it look like in your eyes? What you see, you become. See the best version of yourself. See yourself *healthy*. See yourself *happy*. See yourself *free*.

Power Thoughts

Every day, I am getting healthier. I am beautiful. I have perfect health. I am enjoying my life. My days are filled with great things. I am a victor not a victim. My mind and my body are one. I am at peace with myself. I see my future, and it looks amazing!

Chapter 5

To Eat or to Not Eat

Up to now, I've talked to you about my mental state while going through my transformation. I've been transparent about my journey—my fears, my failures, and my successes. I've done so with the hope of inspiring you to reach your goals as it relates to weight loss. But I wanted to be unique in my approach. I wanted to deal with more than the dos and don'ts we find in so many self-help books abroad.

My challenge has been to help you explore the mental science of weight loss. How you have to win the battle in your mind first. Then results will follow.

Prayerfully, we've done that successfully! Now let's talk food. I'm sure you've heard the cliché, "You are what you eat." I totally agree with that statement. Your body conforms to your treatment of it, so if you consistently succumb to an unhealthy eating regimen, you will be unhealthy. I have learned, and I'm still learning, the art of eating right. Eating more of what's good for me and less of what's not so good has sent my health soaring in the right direction. I no longer crave most wrong food choices. Eating out is a luxury now, not an everyday binge. I've weaned myself off medications simply by policing what I ingest. So let's get to it.

First, you have to know what foods work best for you. Find out your blood type. Certain foods work best for certain blood types. For me, vegetables are best for me and dairies are worse for me. To give a few examples, I had to find a happy median like sugar-free, non-dairy treats, or kale and other green veggies.

Regardless of my food choices, my three absolutes had to always be present. Low sodium, low sugar (turbinado), and water. I specifically avoid refined foods.

Breads, Grains, and Pastas

Make the shift to organic and whole foods. I avoid breads with sugar in them. Imagine my shock to find out the 100 percent whole-wheat bread I thought was healthy was hosting the ingredient that was making me gain weight— sugar, labeled as fructose. Read the ingredients, folks! There are breads, even wheat breads, that are sugar free.

I love pasta and creamy sauces! Yummy! I found organic, sugar-free pastas. I also recently found veggie pasta that is absolutely delicious. Oatmeal is my favorite breakfast choice, but I also like grits and Malt-O-Meal. I cook and season or sweeten to taste, always measuring my sugar and salt intakes. If I eat box cereal, I select the ones with single-digit grams of sugar, and I drink almond milk (remember dairy isn't my friend). I eat brown rice, pinto beans, peas, etc. Again, your food choice may be different. Eat right for your body type.

Snacks

Sometimes, I eat an occasional bag of chips or a chocolate-chip cookie, or a slice of cheesecake; but I do so in moderation. My favorite snack choice is blue corn chips (salt free) with guacamole.

Fruits and Nuts

My fruit choices vary. I love cherries. I found that cherries help reduce belly fat and increase melatonin. Cranberries are one of my favorites too. I also love every nut known to man especially cashews and almonds. I eat them salt free and in healthy, organic trail mixes. There are so many health benefits to eating nuts. I love snacking on them during the day. I encourage you to research whatever your favorite is and see the results for yourself.

For example, almonds are rich in vitamin E, calcium, magnesium, and potassium. They are a good source of protein and fiber. They assist in weight loss. You see, eating the foods you love should be a healthy choice as well.

Vegetables

I love vegetables. Almost every kind. I lean heavily toward green leafy veggies such as greens, kale, cabbage. I'm an onion and bell pepper fanatic! I buy my vegetables raw or frozen. I rarely buy canned foods because of the preservative contents. In my opinion, eating more vegetables than meat or pastas is a slam-dunk to weight loss.

Meats

I look for the following words on the meat packages I buy for my family: no preservatives, cage-free, etc. I eat chicken and fish mostly. If I eat deli meat, I choose the ones with the lowest sodium amounts. I eat but limit my beef intake. Red meat is the hardest to digest for me. If I buy hot dogs, they are 100 percent beef. Tuna is a favorite also. Salmon is another. Again, these are foods that I love. I just learned how to cook and eat from home.

The main point I'm making is this: pay attention to what you're eating. Pay attention to what your children are eating. We can prevent childhood obesity and health decline simply by monitoring the food selections we chose. I know pulling up to a fast-food restaurant is inevitable. However, it shouldn't be our everyday way of life. We can and should live long, healthy, vibrant lives. Be very selective in your food choices. The better your food choices, the less food you'll have to restrict from your diet. Remember, it's a lifestyle change you're shooting for.

Your body will treat you the way you treat it. Stay attuned with your body. Drink plenty of water. Exercise daily. Five minutes is better than zero. Apply the principles I shared with you in this book to your everyday routine. You can and will maintain a healthy body weight. I am living proof!

My Secret Weapon

We talked earlier about the importance of good digestive health. Probiotics have been a life changer for me. I never realized all the health benefits of making sure your diet consisted of a daily dose of them. Probiotics help with healthy digestion, and they help your immune system. I can honestly say that when I constantly included probiotics in my daily routine, I felt better. My digestion was regular. I felt better day after day.

So whether it's yogurt or some all-natural supplement, be sure to maintain a diet filled with probiotics. There are a lot of health benefits of probiotics. I encourage you to research them.

Chapter 6

Brand-New You— How Does It Feel?

For thou, LORD, hast made me glad through thy work: I will triumph in the works of thy hands.

—Psalm 92:4, KJV

This verse sums up the sentiment of how I feel. Throughout my journey, which is ongoing, by the way, my husband would ask me, "Babe, how do you feel?" Remember, I stated from the beginning you have to begin with the end in mind. You have to see it in your mind before you see it in the present. You have to accept as "truth" that it's already yours. You've already lost the weight. Remember the "I am" affirmations we talked about? Said all of that in order to say that I had to answer my husband the right way. I had to say what I wanted even when it didn't seem like it would be so. I had to see and say my desired outcome. Get it?

So I'd answer, "I'm great, honey," or "I feel great." Fear would try to whisper to me, "You're lying." But I would quickly counteract those negative thoughts with the truth. My faith in God's Words over my own thoughts is what I mean. I would speak his truth when my truth was hazy. Eventually, his truth became my reality! When I was weak, he increased my strength.

You have to say it until you see it! I'm not at a loss for words. I'm intentionally saying the same thing over and over again!

This is it! Your secret weapon. Say what you want over and over again until you believe it! Say it in the present tense. Use your "I am" affirmations. Here are a few that worked for me:

- I am healthy!
- I am in great shape!
- I am strong enough to achieve my goal
- I am so attractive to others. They are asking me how I did it!
- Today is a great day!
- I am so grateful for my blessings
- I look forward to helping others

> We, having the same spirit of faith, according as it is written, I believed, and therefore have I spoken; we also believe, and therefore speak.
>
> —2 Corinthians 4:13, KJV

Give yourself permission to be happy! Take yourself to the place of how it feels to lose your desired weight. Everyone's desire is different. So again, don't compare yourself to anyone else. Remember, your words have power. Whatever you say over and over, you will believe.

You Deserve Your Best Self

I've seen a lot of people with great testimonials of weight loss. They didn't all lose weight using the same products or doing the same things. But the one thing they all had in common was the feeling of completeness. That remarkable feeling of completing your goal, your mission. Obtain your heart's desire. As I write this book, I think of how it really feels to win! Think of all the past victories you've had. This one will trump them all. You deserve it!

Never allow anyone to taint your vision of yourself. See yourself healthy. See yourself whole. What you see, you will become. Embrace the real you. The *you* everyone needs to see. At first, things will be awkward. Then your new regimen will be mechanical. But after a while, it will be natural. That's the formula:

Awkward + Mechanical = Natural

I can't stress it enough. Victory is yours. Focus on your "why," not the "how." The "why" will trigger your subconscious to figure out the "how." Take a look at some of my before-and-after shots.

Show and Tell

This is my show-and-tell chapter. Real short and to the point. I've always been a very visual person. My hope is to inspire you to do the same. Do a lot of before-and-after photos of yourself. Someone needs to hear your story. Take a look at some of my before-and-after pictures.

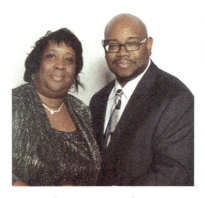
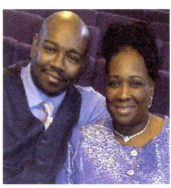

January 2016   August 2016

In seven months, I had lost over seventy pounds. The photo on the right went viral. I remember that when I placed them side by side, I was amazed!

The sense of accomplishment is infectious. It feels good to inspire others to reach their goals and dreams.

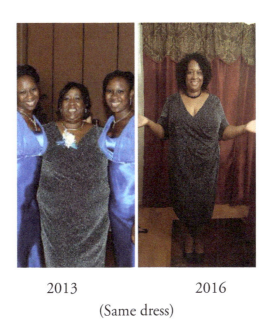

2013   2016
(Same dress)

I'm in tears every time I look at the pictures above. To see where I was three years prior. Even more so where I am currently.

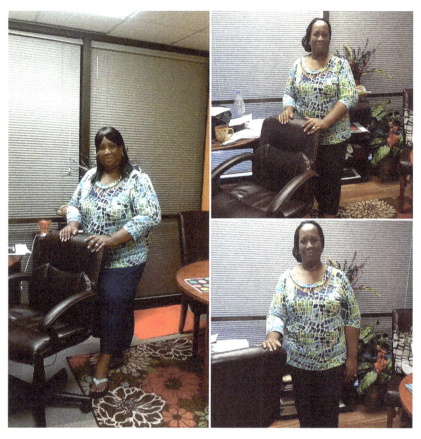

October 2015　　　　　　　August 2016

Now this one (left) was when I had lost a little weight. I had made a little progress from 2013 to 2015, but my real breakthrough came in 2016.

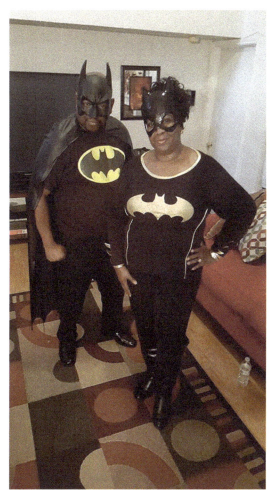

Never in a million years did I believe I'd wear a costume.

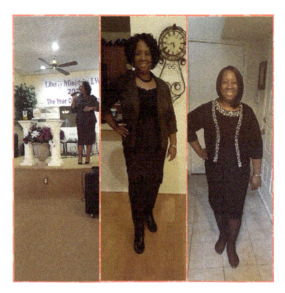

Size 14
How does it feel? It feels absolutely amazing!

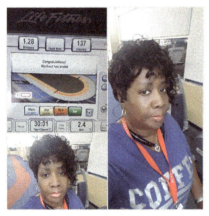 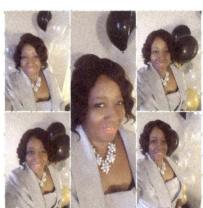

Working out!   Fiftieth Birthday

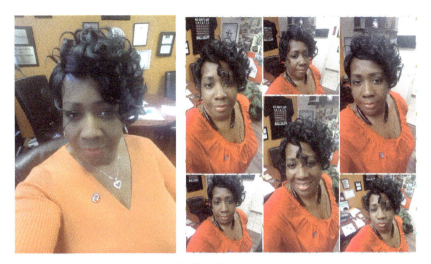

Selfie Queen

I pray this book was inspirational to all who read it. The *losing battle* is not one that we lose. It's one that we *win*!

About the Author

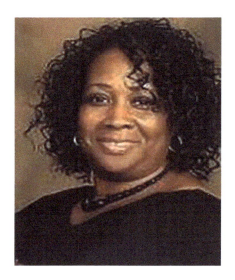

A native of Louisiana, Robertrese Allen is a wife, mother, minister, and business woman. She is passionate about God's people being all that he created them to be.

Co-pastoring Liberty Ministries Family Worship Center in Lancaster, Texas, with her husband, Theodore, as well as running their family business, Robertrese strives to empower God's people to live a victorious life both through knowledge of the Word and through practical concepts and teachings.

Robertrese has been married for thirty-one years to her husband, Pastor Theodore Allen Jr. Together, they have four children and two grandchildren.

CPSIA information can be obtained
at www.ICGtesting.com
Printed in the USA
LVHW01s0824091018
592788LV00013B/800/P